YOUR KNOWLEDGE HAS VALUE

AF141813

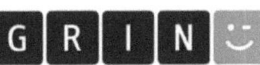

Dr. Peter Ubah Okeke

Platelet Count and Indices of Mean Platelet Volume, Platelet Distribution Width and Platelet Large Cell Ratio - Is there any Sex Difference?

GRIN Publishing

Bibliographic information published by the German National Library:

The German National Library lists this publication in the National Bibliography; detailed bibliographic data are available on the Internet at http://dnb.dnb.de .

Imprint:

Copyright © 2012 GRIN Verlag, Open Publishing GmbH
Print and binding: Books on Demand GmbH, Norderstedt Germany
ISBN: 978-3-656-16569-9

This book at GRIN:

http://www.grin.com/en/e-book/191552/platelet-count-and-indices-of-mean-platelet-volume-platelet-distribution

GRIN - Your knowledge has value

Since its foundation in 1998, GRIN has specialized in publishing academic texts by students, college teachers and other academics as e-book and printed book. The website www.grin.com is an ideal platform for presenting term papers, final papers, scientific essays, dissertations and specialist books.

Visit us on the internet:

http://www.grin.com/

http://www.facebook.com/grincom

http://www.twitter.com/grin_com

PLATELET COUNT AND INDICES OF MEAN PLATELET VOLUME, PLATELET DISTRIBUTION

WIDTH AND PLATELET LARGE CELL RATIO –IS THERE ANY SEX DIFFERENCE?

BY

PETER UBAH OKEKE

March, 2012

Table of contents

Aims and Objectives

The study aimed at investigating platelet count, MPV, PDW and P-LCR profiles as a diagnostic indices for thrombocytopenia and investigate sex differences.

Key words : Platelet count, MPV, PDW, P-LCR,

Acknowledgement

I use this opportunity to thank my beloved wife Mrs Ijeoma Anazali Okeke for her support throughout my program at Atlantic International University Hawaii. My gratitude goes to the entire academic department of Atlantic International University (AIU), our able academic dean Dr. Franklin Valcin, Dr. Jose Mercado, Lee Roobles and Dr. Gonzalez for their immense efforts in making AIU degree programs challenging, conducive, dynamic and reputability in all ramifications.

Many thanks to my academic advisors and teachers like Linda Collazo, Dr. Edgar Colon, Mrs Erica Smith and Dr. Igor Bondarenko for their guidance, advice, correction and prompt communication throughout my program at AIU. Please do not relent in teaching your students that which is profitable internationally , remember that all your tireless efforts are never forgotten.

Abstract

Platelet counts and its associated indices of MPV, PDW and P-LCR were assayed in a total sample of 98 blood donors aged 19 to 55years here in Porto Novo. Among whom 47 were men(47.96%) and 51 were women (52.04%). The mean platelets count of 218.90×10^9/L were recorded among men samples while Platelet count of 247.8×10^9/L were recorded among women blood donors. The platelet count were slightly higher in women than men and this increase is not statistically significant (P=0.01). The indices of platelets, MPV, PDW and P-LCR were also variable among both men and women, again these are not statistically significant (P=0.01).

Conclusion: The present study showed that platelet count are gender dependent and platelet indices should be paid attention to when diagnosing thrombocytopenia. The routine hematologic autoanalyzers should incorporate reticulated platelet absolutely necessary for the accurate assessment of marrow response to thrombocytopenia.

Key words : Platelet count, MPV, PDW, P-LCR,

Corresponding Author: Peter Ubah Okeke

School of Sciences & Engineering

Atlantic International University

www.aiu.edu

Introduction

Platelets are anucleate blood cells that circulate at 150,000 to 450,000/mm3 with mean counts slightly higher in women than men Butkiewicz AM et al (2005). Platelets trigger primary hemostasis on exposure to physical and fluid stimulants that are associated with blood vessel injury. On a wright stained wedge preparation blood film, platelets are distributed through a monolayer at 7 to 21 per 100 × field and have an average diameter of 2.5μm, corresponding to a mean platelet volume(MPV) of 8 to 10 Fl in a direct preparation as determined by laboratory profiling instruments, Tsiara S et al(2003). The internal structure of platelets are complex and is scarcely visible using light microscopy.

Platelets arise from unique bone marrow cells called megakaryocytes. Megakaryocytes are among the largest cells in the body and are polyploidy. In healthy intact bone marrow tissue, megakaryocytes cluster in the extravascular compartment adjacent to the abluminal face of venous sinusoid endothelial cells Lichtman MA et al (1978). Other hematopoietic cells may cross the megakaryocyte cytoplasm to reach the sinusoid lumen, a faux phagocytosis called emperopolesis, Breton-Gorius J (1981). Megakaryocytes also are harvested from the lungs Pedersen NT(1974).

Megakaryocyte Progenitors

The hematopoietic stem cell named the colony forming unit granulocyte, erythrocyte, megakaryocyte, monocytes (CFU-GEMM) differentiates to the megakaryocyte lineage under the influence of hormone thrombopoietin(TPO) and a series of cytokines. There are three megakaryocyte lineage committed progenitor stages, defined by their culture colony characteristics. In order of differentiation, these are the burst forming unit (BFU-meg), colony forming unit(CFU-meg) and the light density CFU(LD-CFU-meg), Cramer EM &Vainchenker W (2006). All three resemble small lymphocytes and cannot be distinguished by wright stained light microscopy. The BFU-meg and CFU-meg are diploid and participate in normal mitosis, maintaining a pool of megakaryocyte progenitors. Their proliferative properties are reflected in their ability to form colonies of hundreds or scores (CFU) of progeny in culture. In contrast to the BFU-meg and CFU-meg, the LD-CFU-meg has little proliferative capacity and produces few cells but progresses to increased nuclear ploidy.

The LD-CFU-meg may be a transitional or promegakaryoblast stage in which polyploidy is established, but the morphology is indistinguishable from small lymphocytes. Megakaryocyte progenitors enter a second developmental compartment, terminal differentiation, as they lose their proliferative capacity.

In specialty laboratories, immunologic probes and flow cytometry are employed to identify megakaryocyte progenitors. Useful megakaryocyte and platelet specific immunologic markers are platelet factor 4 (PF4), von Willebrand Factor (vWF) and platelet glycoproteins Ib (CD42b) and IIb/IIIa (CD41), Cramer EM & Fontenay M(2006). Platelet peroxidase, localized in the endoplasmic reticulum of progenitors and megakaryoblasts also may be identified by cytochemical stain in transmission electron microscopy. Identical peroxidase activity is localized to the dense tubular system of mature platelets, George JN & Colman RW (2006).

Terminal Megakaryocyte Differentiation

Megakaryocyte progenitors leave the proliferative phase and enter terminal differentiation, where they are identified and staged using wright stained morphology in the bone marrow aspirate films or histologically by hematoxylin and eosin (H&E) stain in bone marrow biopsy sections. Past the LD-CFU-meg , there is no further mitosis, but three to four morphologically identifiable stages. Most hematologists use the terms MK I for megakaryoblast, MK II for promegakaryocyte and MK III for megakaryocyte, whereas others add a postmature MK IV stage characterized by a multilobed, highly condensed nucleus.

The MK I cannot be reliably distinguished from the myeloblast or pronormoblast on the basis of routine wright stained morphology of bone marrow aspirates with light microscopy. The microscopist can see plasma membrane blebs, blunt projections that resemble platelets or nuclear lobulation that reflects polyploidy; megakaryoblasts have a greater diameter than the other two blasts on average. Immunologic probes are often needed for definitive identification, the MK I may be identified using immunologic probes for the more differentiated membrane structures (CD42), GP IV (CD36), or mpl, which stands for the TPO receptor site. Immunological probes also may label cytoplasmic fibrinogen and vWF in α-granules.

Light microscopy aside, the MK I possesses most of the ultrastructure associated with the MK II and MK III stages and with platelets. The nucleus, although essentially round, reaches its fully ploidy at the MK I stage. The cytoplasm possesses α- granules and the demarcation system (DMS). The DMS, a series of membrane lined channels invades from the plasma membrane and grows over the course of terminal differentiation to subdivide the entire cytoplasm. MK III is the largest cell in the bone marrow easily detected with the 10 × objective. The nucleus is intensely lobulated and the chromatin is variably condensed. The cytoplasm is eosinophilic, granular, and platelet-like, owing to the through spread of the DMS and α-granules. The MK III is the stage from which platelet shedding or thrombopoiesis proceeds.

Endomitosis

Megakaryocyte maturation is marked by a mysterious form of mitosis that lacks telophase and cytokinesis. This is refered to as endoreduplication or endomitosis, DNA synthesis proceeds to the production of 8N, 16N, or 32N ploidy with completely duplicated sets of chromosomes but no cell division. Some megakaryocytes reach 128N, although this level of ploidy may signal hematologic disease.

A single megakaryocyte may release 2000 to 4000 platelets. The search is ongoing for the molecular basis of endomitosis a cell cycle adaptation found in no other human cell. Just as mitosis ends at the progenitor stage, endomitosis is complete at MK I. The segmentation of the MK II and MK III nucleus probably reflects endomitosis in general, but the degree of duplication is not proportional to lobularity. Ploidy levels are measured easily using mepacrine a nucleic acid dye, in megakaryocyte flow cytometry, Choi ES et al (1995).

Thrombopoiesis

One cannot find reliable evidence for platelet budding or shedding by examining megakaryocytes in situ, even in well structured bone marrow biopsy preparations. In cultured megakaryocytes examined by transmission electron microscopy, the DMS dilates, longitudinal bundles of tubules form, cytoplasmic extensions called proplatelet processes extend and transverse constrictions appear throughout the processes. The proplatelet processes pierce through or between sinusoid lining endothelial cells extend into the venous blood and release platelets. Sometimes whole megakaryocytes escape the marrow in this fashion to lodge in other organs, such as the lungs. Microscopists presume that thrombopoiesis leaves behind naked megakaryocyte nuclei to be consumed by marrow macrophages, although these are rarely seen in bone marrow aspirate films. Their absence leads a few microscopists to think that the lung is the primary site of thrombopoiesis, Levine RF et al (19939.

Hormones and Cytokines of Megakaryocytopoiesis

Thrombopoietin (TPO) is a 70 kilo Dalton molecule with 23% homology to erythropoietin. The messenger RNA for TPO has been found in the liver, kidney and smooth muscle cells. TPO is primarily produced in the liver and is the ligand that binds to a megakaryocyte and platelet membrane receptor protein, mpl. McDonald TP (1992) reported that TPO induces stem cells to differentiate into megakaryocyte progenitors in synergy with cytokines which further induces differentiation of megakaryocyte progenitors to megakaryocytes and inturn induces the proliferation and maturation of megakaryocytes. Recombinant TPO in several forms elevates the platelet counts in healthy blood donors and in patients treated for a variety of neoplasms, including acute leukemia and has shown some promise in clinical trials, Kuter DJ & Begley CG (2002).

Cell- derived stimulators of megakaryocytopoiesis include interleukin(IL)-3, IL-6 and IL-11. Interleukin-3 seems to act in synergy with TPO to induce early differentiation of stem cells whereas IL-6 and IL-11 act in the presence of TPO to enhance the later act of endomitosis, megakaryocyte maturation and platelet release. IL-11 has been synthesized and used to stimulate platelet production in chemotherapy induced thrombocytopenia, Demetri GD (2001). Other cytokines and hormones that participate synergistically with TPO and the interleukins are stem cell factor; also called kit ligand or mast cell growth factor; granulocyte macrophage colony stimulating factor; granulocyte colony stimulating factor and erythropoietin.

PF-4, β-thromboglobulin, neutrophil activating peptide 2, IL-8 and other factors inhibit in-vitro megakaryocyte growth which indicates they may have a role in the control of megakaryocytopoiesis invivo. Internally, reduction in the transcription factors FOG, GATA-1 and NF-E2 diminish megakaryocytopoiesis at the progenitor, endomitosis and terminal maturation phases, Chang M et al (2003).

Platelets

The proplatelet process sheds platelets , cells consisting of granular cytoplasm with a membrane but no nuclear material into the venous sinus. Their diameter in the monolayer of a wright stained peripheral blood wedge films averages 2.5μm. Mean platelet volume as measured in an isotonic suspension flowing through the detector cell of a clinical laboratory instrument ranges from 8 to 10FL. A frequency distribution of platelet volume is log- normal, indicating a subpopulation of large platelets.

Ault KA (1993) stated that reticulated platelets or stress platelets appear in compensation for thrombocytopenia. Reticulated platelets are markedly larger than ordinary mature circulating platelets, their diameter in blood films exceeding 6μm and their MPV reaching 12 to 14 FL, Briggs C et al (2004). Platelet count is an integral component of the full blood count. Unexpectedly, abnormal platelet counts are sometimes obtained in clinical setting. For example a false low platelet count could be due to platelet aggregation which can be easily picked up on a blood film examination by the technologist. Failure to recognize this phenomenon has sometimes led to a serious error misdiagnosis of a patient as suffering from idiopathic thrombocytopenic Purpura (ITP) and has led to corticosteroid therapy and even splenectomy in one case reported by Pegels JG et al (1982).

Before any clinical decision on diagnosis or management of the patient is made, the abnormal platelet count has to be validated. In interpreting the platelet count result, it is very important to understand the physiological and various technical factors that could affect the platelet count such as the method of collecting blood specimen, preparation of the platelet sample, the type of instrument and the calibration method used.

Normal Platelet count

The normal range of platelet count is 150,000 to 450,000 /mm^3 and this range in health remains constant, physiological variables affecting the platelet count have to be considered when commenting on the results of the platelet count. Dacie and Lewis (2006) reported no age differences at birth and in the first few weeks of infancy, however, the platelet count tends to bat the lower level of the adult normal range and rising to adult levels at about 6 months. However, Novak RW and co-workers (1987) found children to have higher platelet count than adults, whereas the practical experience of Stevens RF and Alexander MK (1977) proved that platelet count are about 20% higher in women than men. Nevertheless, the early experiment of Morley A (1969) considered that platelet count may fall in normal women at about the time of menstruation and there is strong evidence of a cycle with a 21 to 35 day rhythm. Caims JW et al (1977) claimed that platelet count fall dramatically during pregnancy while Giles C (1981) who worked extensively on the platelet count and its mean platelet volume argued that if subjects with pregnancy related hypertension are excluded, no fall is observed.

The method of collecting blood influences the platelet count. The paper presented by Tai et al (1995) stated that capillary blood obtained by finger prick generally has lower platelet count than venous puncture. This was also vindicated by the early conclusion of Brecher G et al (1953) that the lower platelet count in capillary blood is probably due to the adhesion of some platelets at the site of the wound and the diluting effect of the tissue fluid, occurring while squeezing the finger. The small amount of blood collected in capillary blood does not allow for a recheck on the same sample if the initial result is doubtful. In clinical laboratory practice, a venous blood sample is preferable and more dynamic, safe and reliable in most laboratory automated instrument. However, capillary blood may be used when there is difficulty during the venous puncture or if the patient requires daily blood count monitoring as in patients with hematological malignancies who are undergoing radiotherapy or chemotherapy.

Ethylene diamine tetra acetic acid(EDTA) is a very convenient anticoagulant to use for routine platelet count, occasionally the presence of EDTA causes the platelets to clump and the count to be falsely low. The platelet agglutinins responsible for this may be IgG or IgM antibodies active in the presence of EDTA. Such antibodies may be optimally active at lower temperature (0-4°c) and the aggregation may be time dependent. Platelet satellitism a well known phenomenon may be formed with adhesion of platelets around the neutrophil.

In the presence of EDTA dependent agglutinins, a repeat platelet count using citrate or heparin as an anticoagulant is necessary for an accurate result. Platelet aggregation may also be due to an antibody acting independently of EDTA. Some of these agglutinins are also cold agglutinins and an accurate result may be produced by warming a fresh sample.

Platelet volume indices are useful in assessing the etiology of thrombocytopenia. In addition, a normal platelet distribution width in the setting of thrombocytosis is highly suggestive of a reactive etiology, Avi Leader et al (2012). Higher MPV is also associated with the presence of cardiovascular risk factors, chest pain due to acute coronary syndrome and adverse outcome after acute coronary syndrome. The calculated Mean Platelet Volume is very dependent on the technique of measurement and on the length and conditions of storage prior to testing the blood. When MPV is measured by impedance technology, it has been discovered to vary inversely with the platelet count in normal subjects. If this curve is extrapolated, it has been found that data fit the extrapolated curve when thrombocytopenia is caused by peripheral platelet destruction; hence, the MPV is lower than predicted when thrombocytopenia is caused by megaloblastic anemia or bone marrow failure, Bessman et al (1982).

Other platelet parameters include the Platelet distribution width (PDW) which is a measure of platelet anisocytosis and the PDW is useful in distinguishing essential thrombocythaemia (PDW increased) from reactive thrombocytosis (PDW normal).

Within the wide normal reference range, there are some ethnic differences and in healthy west Indians and Africans, platelet count may on the average be 10% to 20% lower than those in Europeans living in the same environment, Bain BJ and Seed M (1986). Allsop P et al (1988) reported that strenuous exercise causes a 30% to 40% increase in platelet count and the mechanism is similar to that which occurs with leucocytes.

Methodology

98 apparently healthy blood donors of both sexes were bled in hospital of Porto Novo, during blood donation sensibilization exercise. The age range of all donors were between 19 to 55 years old, platelet count and its index were assayed within 20 minutes of blood collection, using sysmex KX21-N autoanalyzer, Control assays were done using eight check - 3wp assay and reference values were as follows;

Platelet count 150 to 450 × 10^9/l

Mean Platelet Volume 7.7 to 11.0 FL

Platelet Distribution Width 6.7 to 8.3 FL

Platelet large cell ratio 4 to 20 %

Platelet Preparation for Automated Counting

Platelets may be prepared in three major ways for automated counting depending on the type of counter used. It can be counted in platelet rich plasma, in whole blood in the presence of intact red cells or in whole blood following lysis of red cells. When platelets are counted in platelet rich plasma, falsely low platelet count may be due to loss of platelets during preparation. Inaccuracy may also be consequent to failure to correct for the platelet free plasma which is trapped in the red cell column. When platelets are counted in whole blood in the presence of red cells, falsely high platelet count may be due to red cells fragments or Microcytic red cells counted as platelets. When platelet count is taken in whole blood following lysis of red cells, falsely high platelet count may be due to the presence of malarial parasites. According to this work, no malaria check is necessary because there is practically no case of malaria in this locality of Cape Verde, other clinical issues that can affect platelet counts include; Howell- Jolly bodies, Heinz bodies, Pappenheimer bodies, erythrocyte debris formed when red cells are aggregated by antibodies or agglutinating paraproteins, Morton BD et al (1980).

Platelet Size Calibration

Most instrument measure cells falling between 2 to 20 femtolitres as platelets. This raw data is plotted on the platelet histogram. While the bulk of the platelet population falls within a fixed threshold, others exist outside these boundaries, microthrombocytes on the low end and macrothrombocytes on the high end. However, cytoplasmic fragment, Microcytic red cells and debris can be included as platelets. To overcome this problem, mathematical curve fitting is applied to the raw data histogram to deliver a more reliable platelet count, therefore eliminating non- platelet particles. The raw data (2-20FL) is tested against a set of criteria and fitted to a log normal curve from 0 to 70 FL. The curve must be positive, the mode must fall between 3 and 15 FL and the coefficient of variation of platelet size or PDW is less than 20%. Once these criteria are met, the autoanalyzer uses the fitted curve to determine the platelet count (equal to area under the curve from 0 to 70 FL). If one of the above criteria is not met, an R flag appears next to platelet count no log normal curve will be fitted.

The platelet count is then derived using the area under the curve of raw data from 2 to 20 FL, which may be less than accurate. In the presence of an instrument flag, the platelet count has to be verified by a peripheral blood film. The setting of the upper threshold of platelet count is less critical with instrument counting on platelet rich plasma as contaminating red cells are not usually present. In instrument such as coulter or sysmex, the application of sweep flow in the counting chamber improves the accuracy of the platelet count. It was found that red cells produced characteristic swirling patterns as they passed through the aperture. They may re-enter the sensing zone and produce small pulses that could be counted as platelets. To prevent this, sweep flow lines carrying diluents are attached to the bottom of the counting chamber. Vaccum pulls the diluents from these lines past the aperture outlets, preventing re-entry of the cells into the sensing zone.

Falsely Low Platelet Count

Falsely low platelet count are more common than falsely high counts. This error is mostly due to partial clotting of the specimen or platelet aggregation. The platelets may form platelet satellitism around the Neutrophils, this is mostly seen in blood samples collected in EDTA. However, proper collection technique and prompt testing will reduce blood clotting and platelet aggregation, Macrothrombocytes may cause falsely low platelet counts as these large platelets will not be counted as they fall outside the upper threshold of platelet calibration.

Falsely High Platelet Count

Microcytic red cells less than 20FL will be counted as platelets and platelet count will be spuriously elevated. The red cell volume and the platelet histogram, together with instrument flag provide clues to this problem. Blast fragments or cytoplasmic fragments of white cells can simulate platelets as well. Presence of cryoglobulin result in pseudothrombocytosis. Correct counts can often be obtained by warming the sample to 37°c. Bacteria in the blood of patients may be counted as platelets leading to high platelet count. In-vitro hemolysis can result in red cell ghosts counted as platelets. However, in whichever case, blood film examination and manual count remains fundamental in the resolution of all these problems.

Statistical Analysis

ANOVA tests were applied for comparing the two groups (Men and Women). ANOVA is another method for the sum of square analysis of variation when comparing two sets of Data. Measurement were compared using F-distribution table at 99% for the appropriate degree of freedom, this serves to clearify whether differences between sets of analysis are significant and not the result of chance alone.

Results

The men category were of age group 20 to 53 years old making 47.96% of those who donated blood on 28th March, 2012 for the platelet and its associated indices and total number of men (n) were 47.

Table 1; Presents the platelet count, MPV, PDW and P-LCR of men category in relation to age group of the 28th March, 2012 blood donation.

Profiles	Age group			
	18-30	31-40	41-50	≥51
Platelet count 10^9/L	148.4	35	25.09	10.34
MPV FL	6.08	3.7	1.31	0.37
PDW FL	7.44	2.43	1.39	0.44
P-LCR %	14.04	5.11	2.89	0.73

Table 2; Presents the platelet count, MPV, PDW, and P-LCR of women category in relation to age group of the 28th March, 2012 blood donation.

Profiles	Age group			
	18-30	31-40	41-50	≥51
Platelet count 10^9/L	154.0	46.4	36.8	10.50
MPV FL	5.9	1.96	1.4	0.34
PDW FL	7.3	2.47	1.9	0.40
P-LCR %	13.2	4.71	3.7	0.62

The women category were of age range 19 to 52 years old with a total number (n) of 51 making 52.04% of the total number of those tested.

Discussion

In this study a total of 98 blood donors were bled among whom 51 were women(52.04%) and 47 were men (47.96%). However, platelet count and its profiles were done in all samples. The mean platelet count of 218.90 $\times 10^9$/L were registered in men category while the mean platelet count of 247.80 $\times 10^9$/L were recorded for the women category. In all age range studied, there was a slight increase in platelet count in women than men, this increase was not statistically significant (P=0.01) in all the platelet indices tested. Also in all the people who donate blood in this region were mainly young adults and the older adults were unlikely to donate blood. Novak RW et al (1987) reported that children have higher platelet count than adults, this cannot be proved in this work because the sample used were all from adult donors.

This study follows similar pattern with other workers that reported higher platelet counts in women than men, Stevens RF & Alexander MK (1977), although in this study the differences were not statistically significant (P=0.01). This reflect different hormonal profiles or compensatory mechanism associated with menstrual blood loss and also proved that platelet count is gender dependent, Anna Butkiewicz et al (2006). The indices of MPV, PDW, and P-LCR in both women and men are also not statistically significant. The MPV is a machine calculated measurement of the average size of platelets found in blood and is typically included in tests as part of the full blood count. Since the average platelet size is larger when the body is producing increased numbers of platelets, the MPV test results can be used to make inferences about platelet production in bone marrow or platelet destruction problems. Abnormally, low MPV values correlate primarily with thrombocytopenia when it is due to impaired production. Although platelet distribution width, platelet large cell Ratio and Mean platelet volume have sufficient sensitivity and specificity in the diagnosis of immune thrombocytopenia, in evaluating the mechanism of thrombocytopenia, it is necessary to know which is more dominant, hypo-productive thrombocytopenia or hyper- destructive thrombocytopenia. In this study, the MPV, PDW and P-LCR showed no observable differences and there is no observable thrombocytopenia in all donors of this study. The controversy related to whether platelets change volume or density in the circulation is still not clearly resolved and although the relationship between platelet number and size and megakaryocyte number, size and ploidy have been well described but the factors that regulate this interaction are still poorly understood.

Conclusion: The present study showed that platelet count are gender dependent and platelet indices should be paid attention to when diagnosing thrombocytopenia. The routine hematologic autoanalyzers should incorporate reticulated platelet absolutely necessary for the accurate assessment of marrow response to thrombocytopenia.

References

Allsop P et al (1988); Does splenic auto transfusion occur during high intensity cycle exercise in man? Journal of Physiology (London) 407:24P

Ault KA (1993); Flow cytometric measurement of platelet function and reticulated platelets. Ann NY Acad Sci 677:293

Bain BJ and Seed M (1986); Platelet count and platelet size in healthy Africans and west Indians. Clinical and Laboratory Hemat 8 :43-45

Bessman et al (1982); Platelet size in health and hematologic disease. American Journal Clinical Path 78:150-153

Breton-Gorius J (1981); On the alleged phagocytosis by megakaryocytes. Br. J Hemato 47:635-636

Brecher G et al (1953); The reproducibility and constancy of the platelet count. Am J Clin Path 23:12-26

Briggs C et al (2004); Assessment of an immature platelet fraction(IPF) in peripheral thrombocytopenia. Br. J Hemat 126:93-99

Butkiewicz AM et al (2005); Platelet count, Mean platelet volume and thrombocytopoietic indices in healthy women and men. Thromb Res 118:199-204

Caims JW et al (1977); Platelet levels in pregnancy. J Clin Path 30:392

Chang M et al (2003); Immune thrombocytopenic Purpura(ITP), plasma and purified ITP monoclonal autoantibodies inhibit megakaryocyopoiesis in-vitro. Blood 102:887-895

Dacie JV and Lewis SM (2006); Reference range and normal values. Practical Hematology eleven eds. UK

Demetri GD (2001); Targeted approaches for the treatment of thrombocytopenia. Oncologist 6(suppl) 5:15-23

Giles C (1981); The platelet count and MPV. Br J Hemat 48:31-7

Kuter DJ and Begley CG(2002); Recombinant human thrombopoietin; basic biology and evaluation of clinical studies. Blood 100:3457-3469

Levine RF et al (1993); Circulating megakaryocytes; delivery of large numbers of intact mature megakaryocytes of the lung. Eur J Hemat 51:233-246

Lichtman MA et al (1978); Parasinusoid allocation of Megakaryocytes in marrow. Am J Hemat 4:303

McDonald TP (1992); Thrombopoietin; its biology, clinical aspects and possibilities. Am J Pediatr Hemat Onco 14:8-21

Morton BD et al (1980); Pappenheimer bodies. An additional cause for a spurious platelet count. Am J Clin Path 74:310-1

Morley A (1969); A platelet cycle in normal individuals. Austral Ann Med 18:127

Novak RW et al (1987); Normal platelet and mean platelet volume in pediatric patients. Lab Med 18:613-4

Pedersen NT (1974); The pulmonary vessels as a filter for circulating megakaryocytes. Scand J Hemat 13:225

Pegels JG et al (1982); Pseudothrombocytopenia: An immunological study on platelet antibodies dependent on EDTA. Blood 59:157-61.

Stevens RF and Alexander MK (1977); A sex difference in the platelet count. Br J Hemat 37:295

Tai YH et al (1995); Comparison of platelet counts in simultaneous venous and capillary blood samples using an automated platelet analyzer. Singapore Med J 36:269-72

Tsiara S et al (2003); Platelets as predictors of vascular risk: Is there a practical index of platelet activity? Clin Appl Thromb Hemost 9:177-190